My Vegetables Book

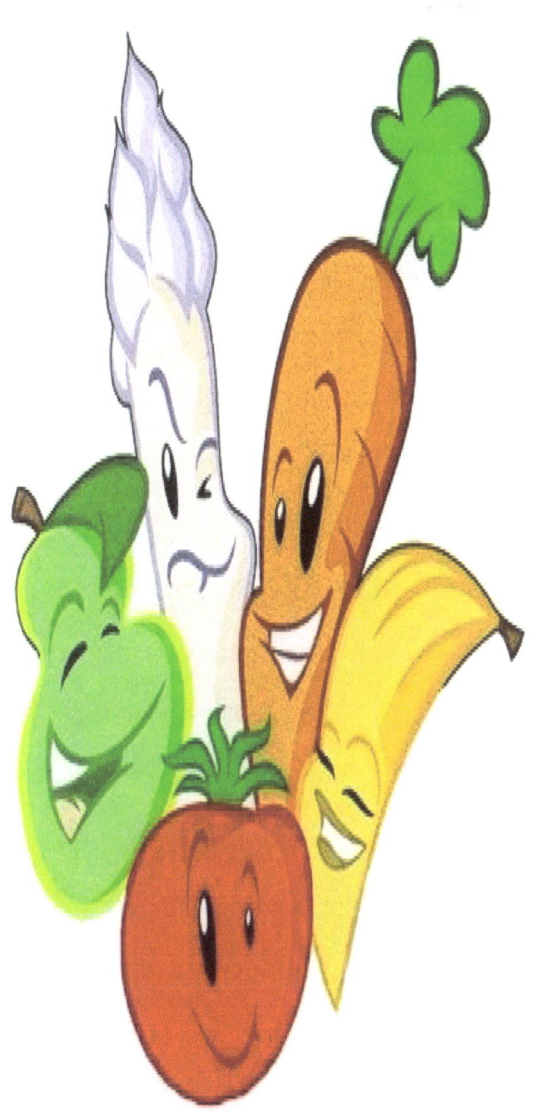

Written By: Melissa L. Bryant

I dedicate this book to my children Lavicia, Vyshonn, Damarius, Darrell and Rashad who I love so much.

I dedicate this book to my nieces Kyrenne and Claudia.

I dedicate this book to my nephews Jarvis, Conner and Amarie.

I dedicate this book to the children at my church Daleville Christian fellowship.

I dedicate this book to all the children around the world.

It's very important that you eat your vegetables boys and girls so you can stay healthy.

Parents you can teach your child or children to identify the vegetables on their plate as they eat it.

Ask them to describe the vegetables on their plate, such as the shape, color, taste and texture.

I use to tell my children that the nutrient found in the vegetables helps our bodies to do the following things like help our skin and eyes.

It also helps keep our digestive tracts healthy so they can be big boys and girls.

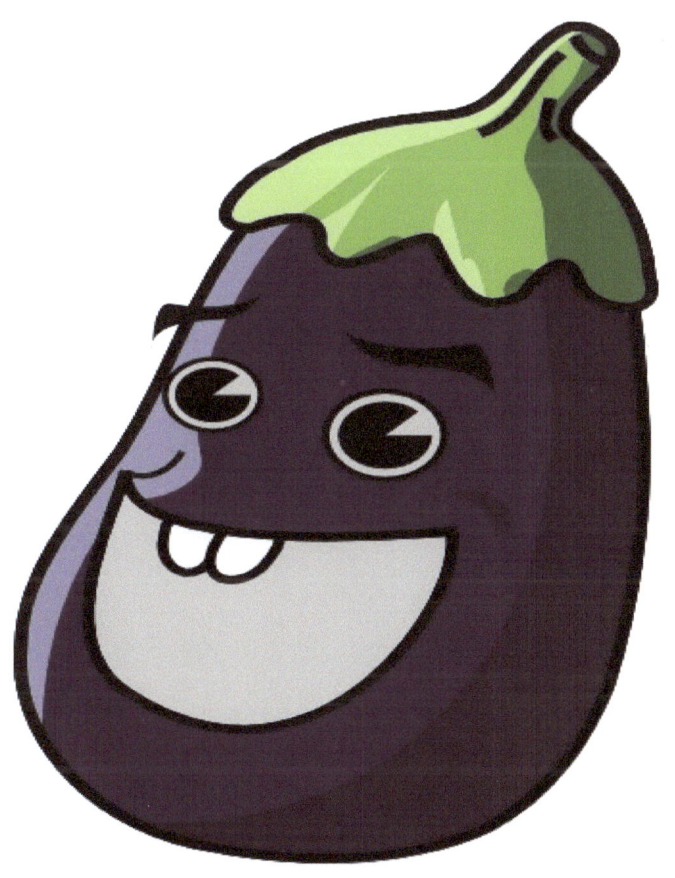

I like eggplant. What about you?

(1)

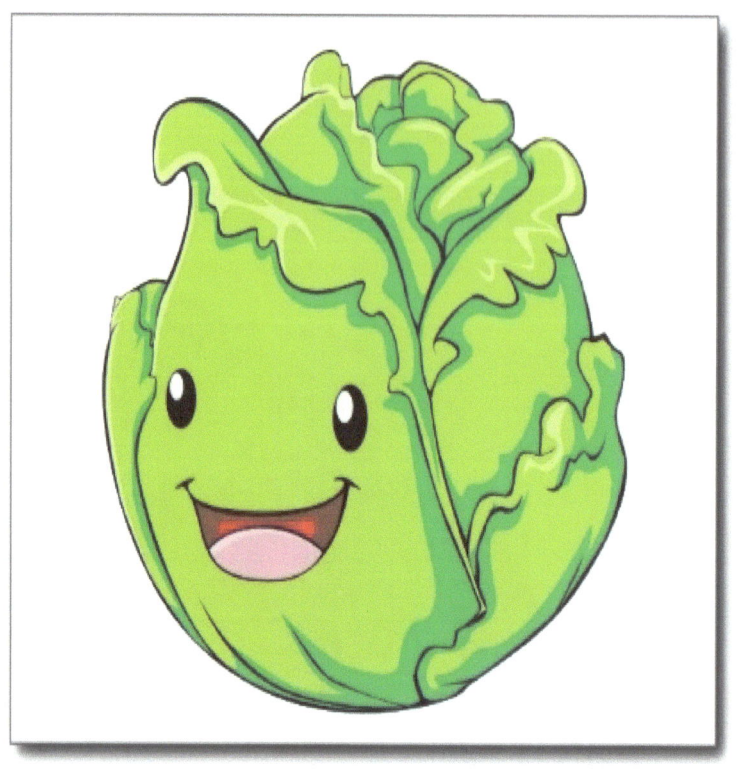

Cabbage is delicious. You should really try it.

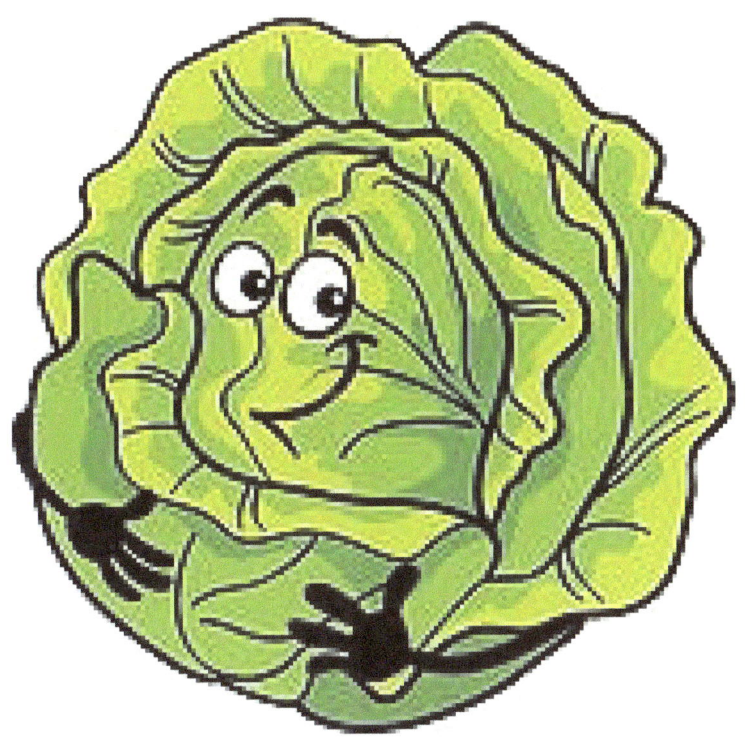

Rabbits eat lettuces. What about you?

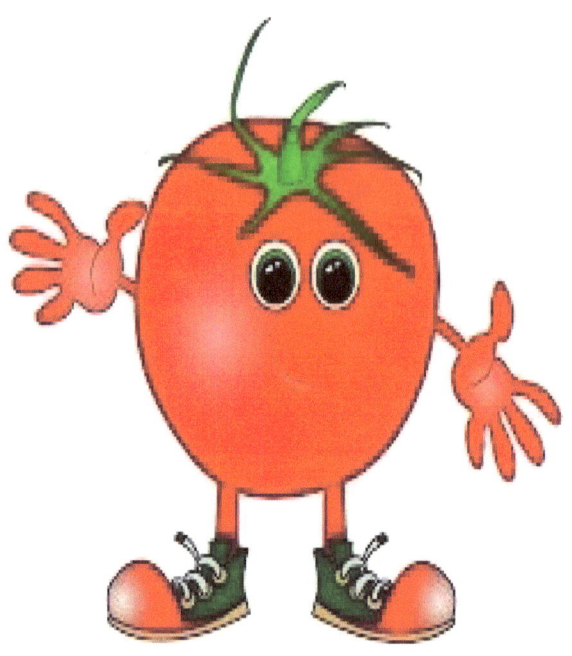

I like tomato. What about you?
Ketchup is made out of tomato.

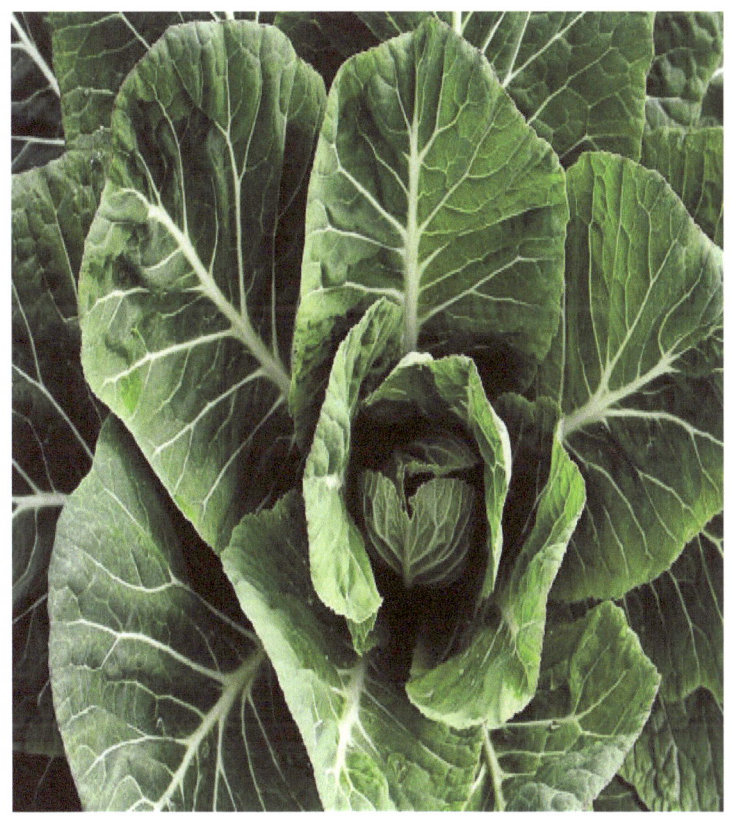

Collard green is my favorite with Turkey meat, rice, and cornbread. You should really try it.

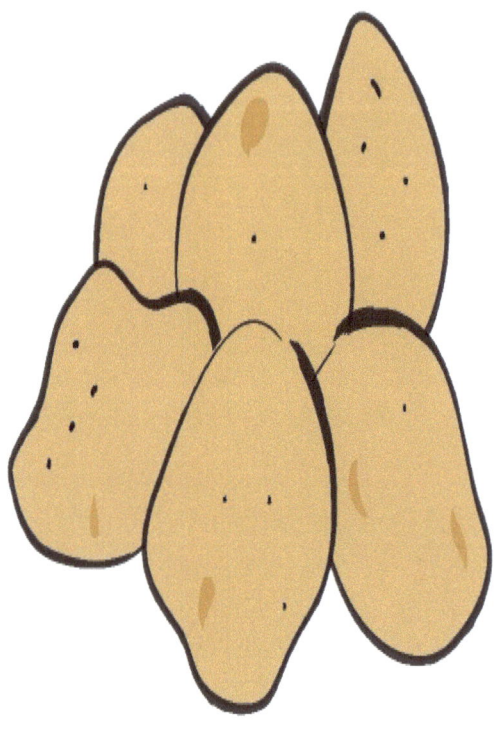

Potatoes are delicious. I love potatoes fries.
What about you?

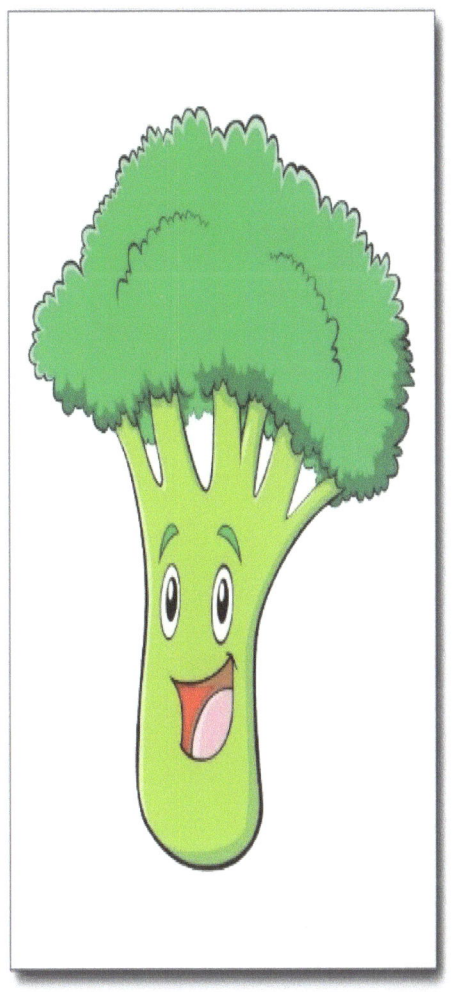

Broccoli is delicious with cheese. You should really try it.

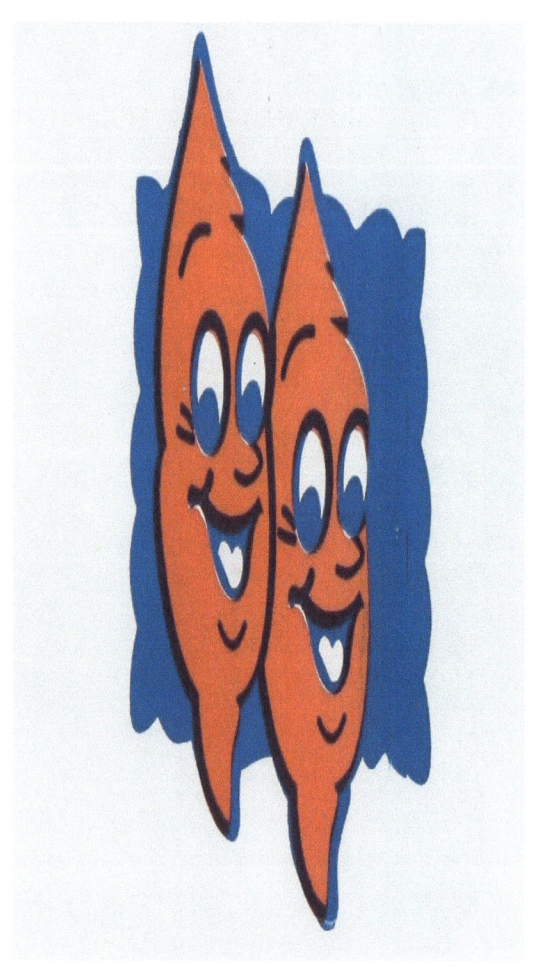

I like yams. What about you?

(8)

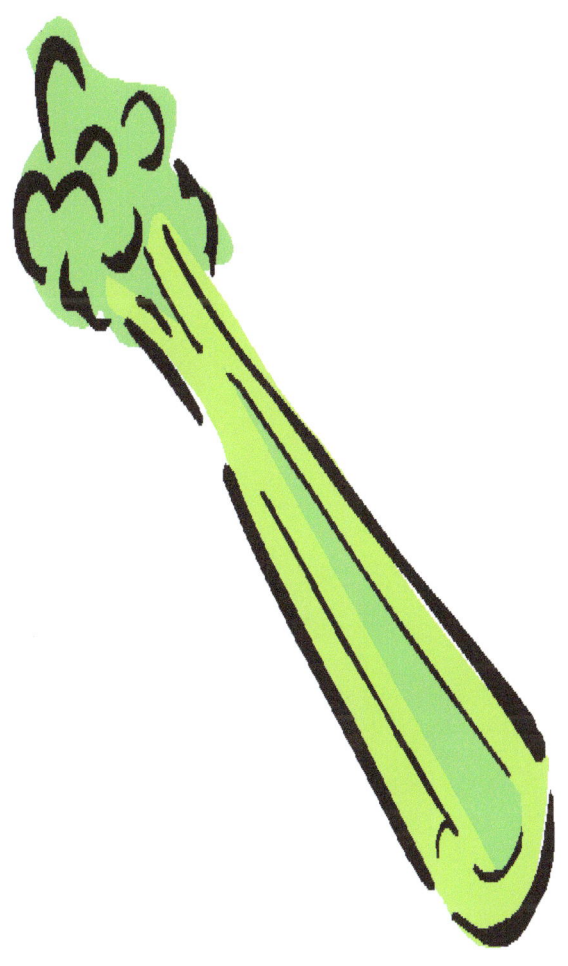

Celery and peanut butter is delicious.
What do you think?

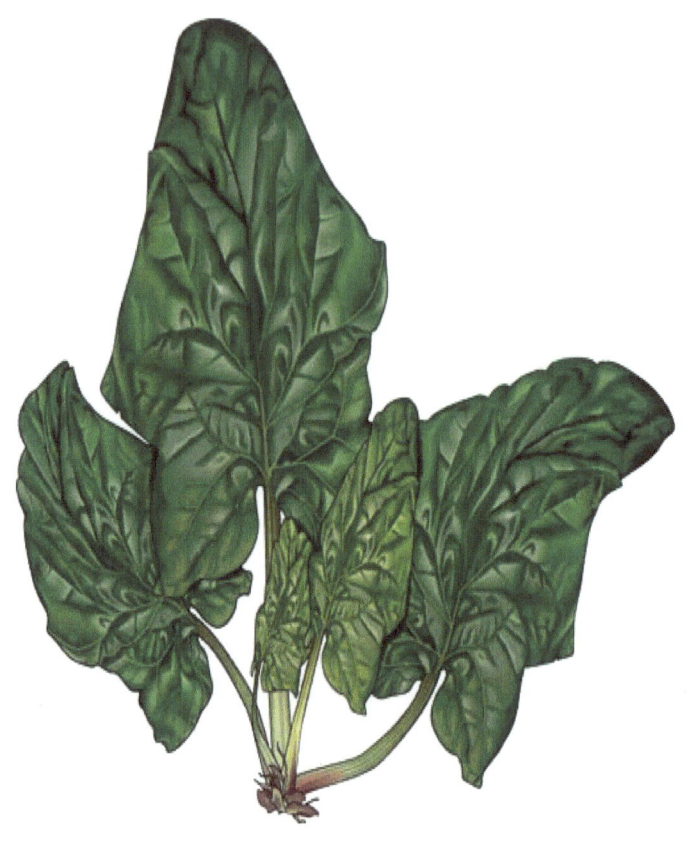

I like spinach. You really should try it.

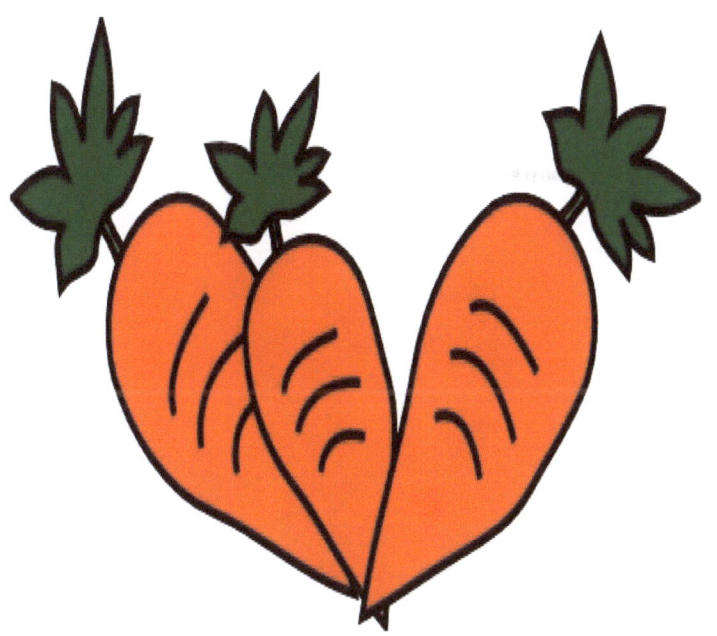

I love carrots with Ranch dressing.
What about you?

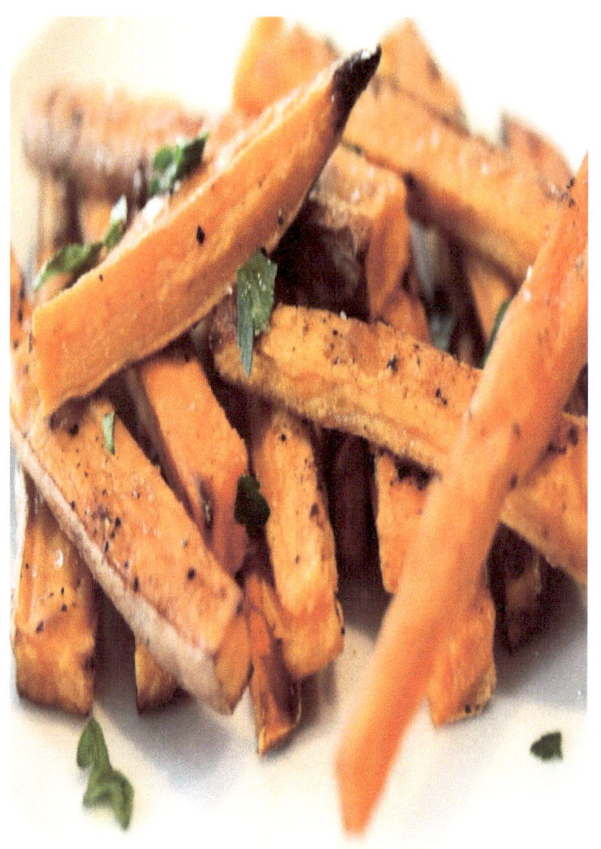

Sweet potatoes fries are delicious. What do you think?

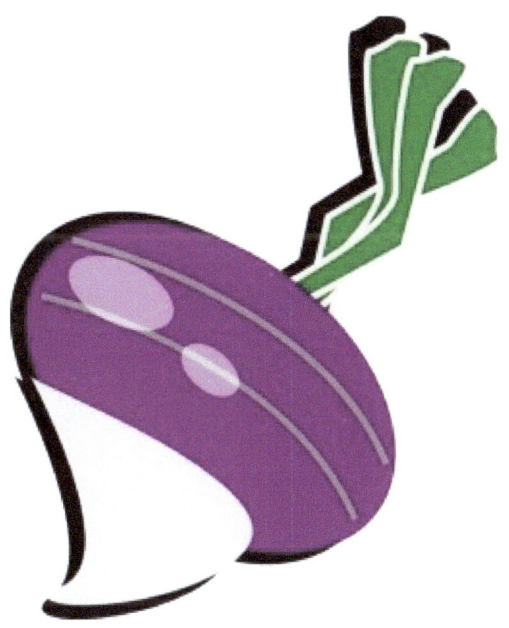

Turnip is delicious. You should really try it.

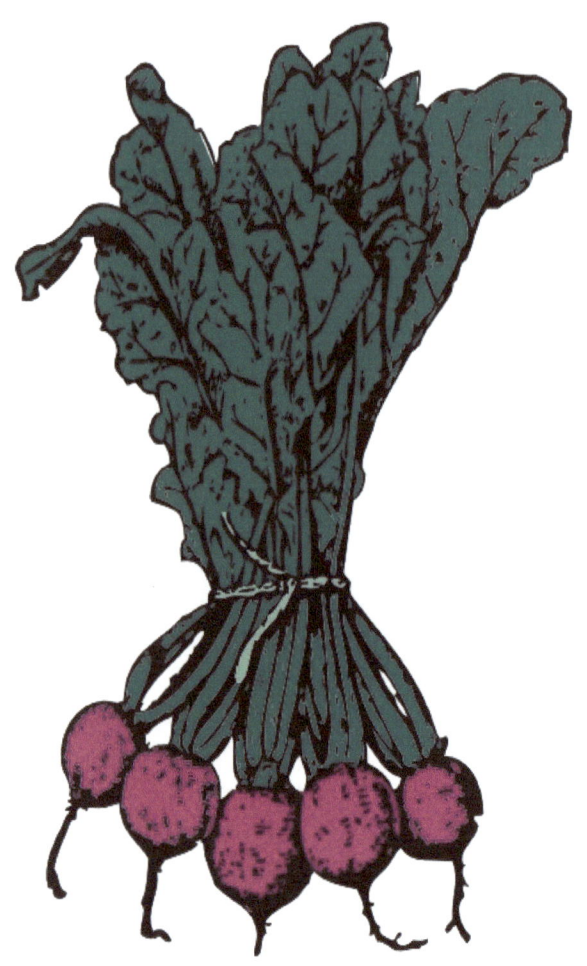

I like beets. What about you?

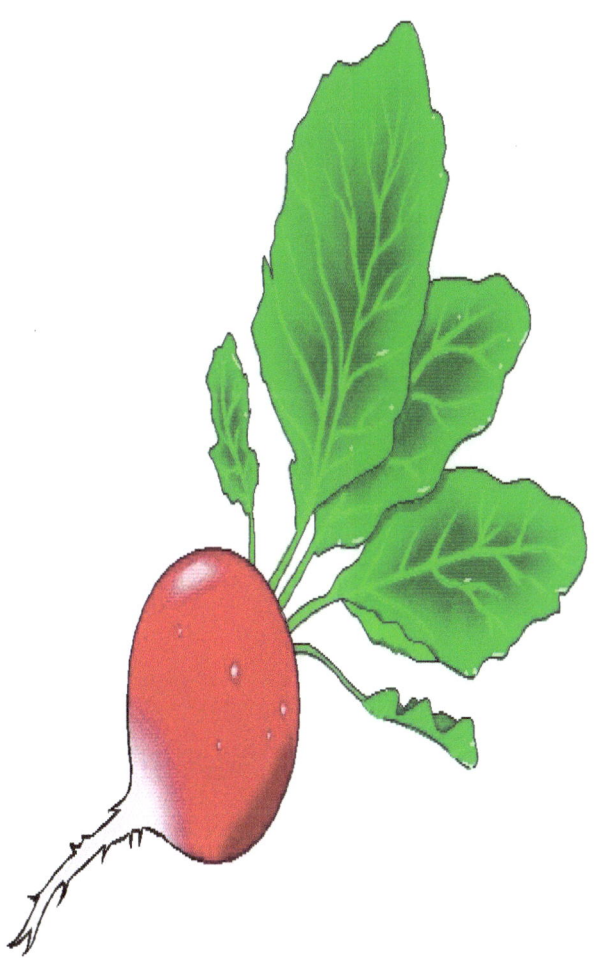

Radish is delicious. You should really try it.

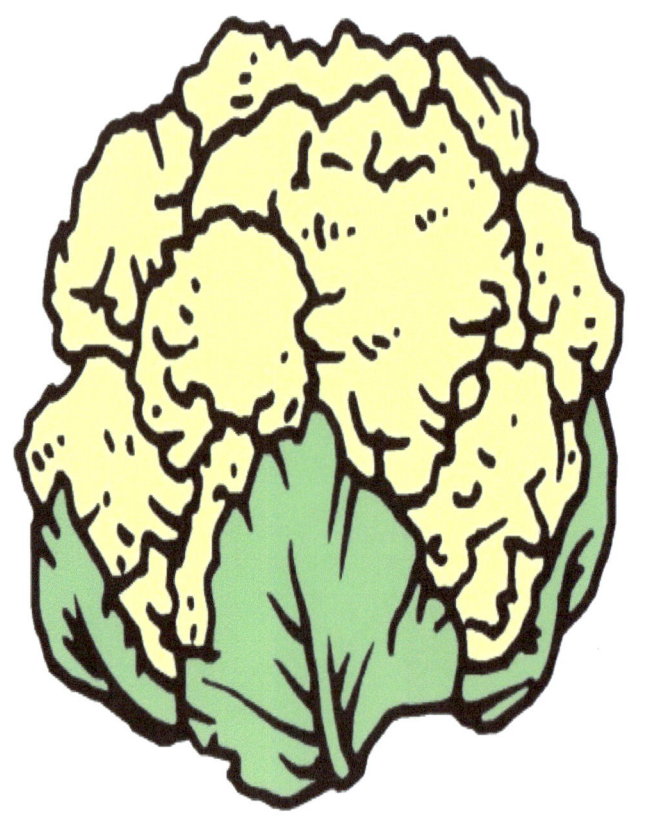

Cauliflower is delicious. What do you think?

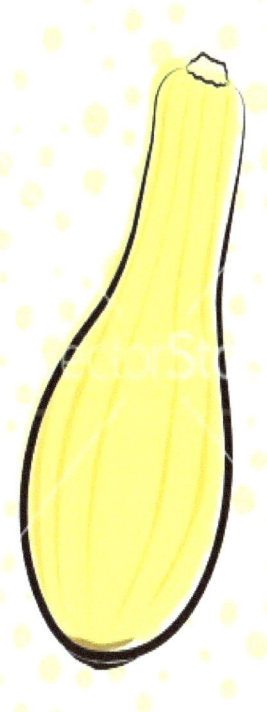

I like yellow squash. What do you think?

(17)

I love a cucumber. What about you?

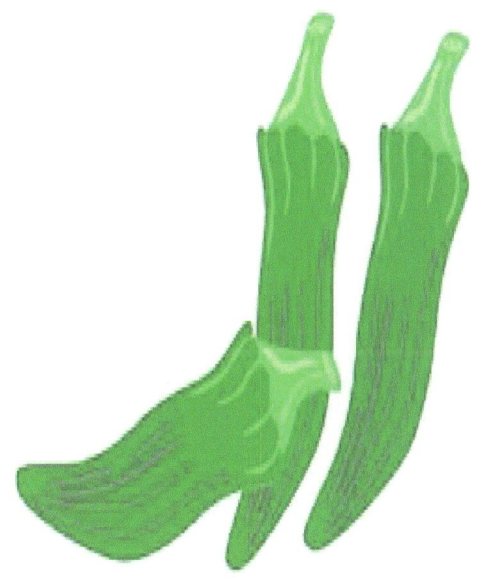

I like green okra. What about you?

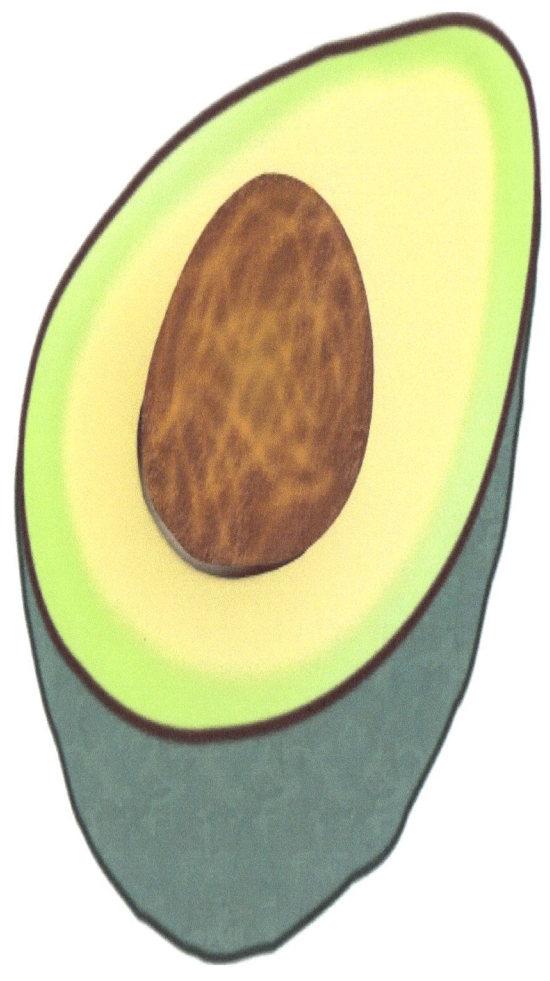

Avocado taste so delicious. You should you try?

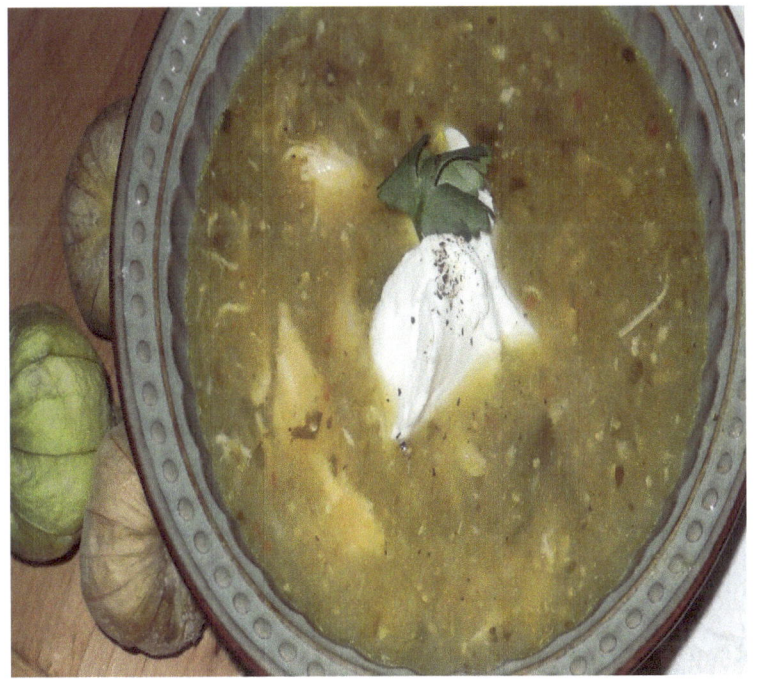

Tomatillos are delicious in soup. What do you think?

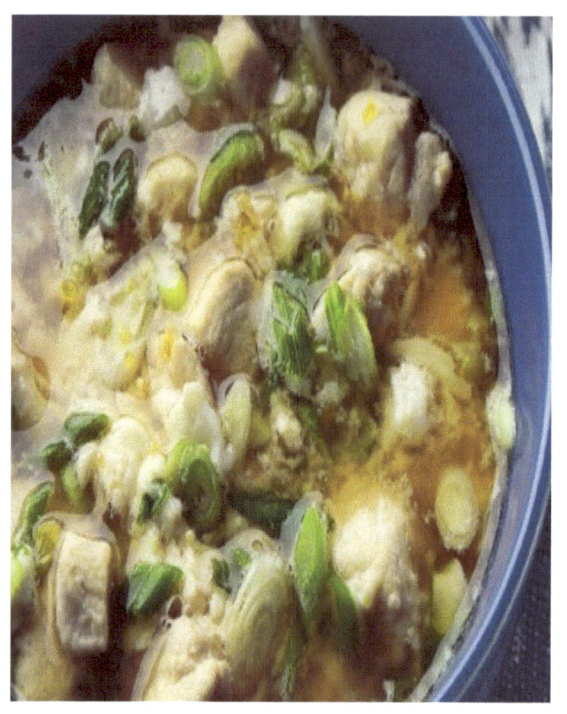

Scallions taste so good in chicken soup.
You should really try it.

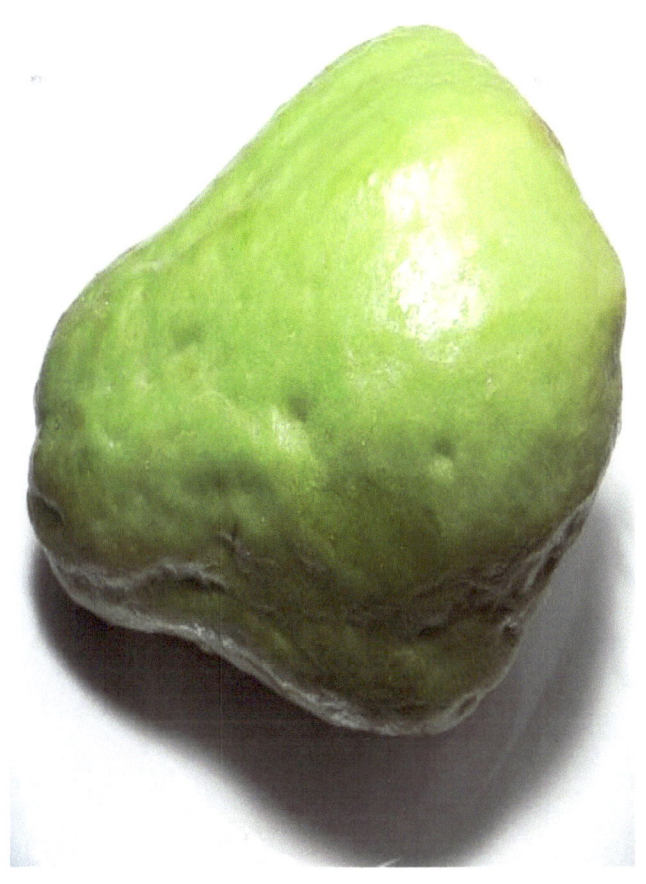

A chayote taste so delicious. You really should try it.